DIABETES WELLNESS: CUSTOMIZED DIET SOLUTIONS

Empower Your Health with Personalized Nutritional Plans for Optimal Diabetes Management

Dr. Harmony Wells

Dr. Harmony Wells

TABLE OF CONTENT

Dr. Harmony Wells

INTRODUCTION

Diabetes is a common and complex illness that affects people all over the world and requires a sophisticated understanding and treatment plan. The variety within this range, from Type 1 to Type 2 diabetes, as well as gestational diabetes, necessitates comprehensive investigation of causes, risk factors, and diagnostic clarity. This trip explores the effects on the body and psyche in addition to elevated blood sugar levels. This investigation concludes with a look toward the future, highlighting the dynamic nature of our knowledge, as we traverse the complex terrain of diabetes, from lifestyle changes to pharmaceuticals. Come along on this trip with us as we reveal the fundamental tactics for successful management, emphasizing the critical role personalized diets play in reaching diabetes wellness.

Diabetes is a spectrum disease, not a singular illness, with each type having special traits and complications of its own. Every type of diabetes requires a complex understanding, including the autoimmune-driven Type 1 diabetes, the lifestyle-related Type 2 diabetes, and the transient gestational diabetes. We'll explore the genetic predispositions, environmental triggers, symptoms, and subtleties of diagnosis that characterize this complex health landscape in this chapter. A key component of the all-

Diabetes wellness: Customized diet solutions

encompassing management of diabetes, nutrition is about much more than just providing for basic needs. It develops into an effective instrument, a regular ally in controlling weight, regulating blood sugar, and promoting general well being. This chapter will examine the vital role that nutrition plays in the intricate dance of glucose regulation. Specifically, it will look at how food choices, meal timing, and meal composition affect glucose regulation.

Let this exploration serve as a guide as we work through the pages that follow, offering advice, techniques, and empowerment to people with diabetes and those who support them. Together, we'll discover the secrets to comprehending the nuances of diabetes and releasing the power of nutrition to promote real wellness as opposed to merely management.

CHAPTER ONE

THE DIABETES LANDSCAPE

Within the broad field of health, diabetes presents as a unique and complex terrain. This complex terrain is formed by a multitude of factors, all of which add to the difficulty of comprehending and treating this condition. Entering the diabetic terrain, we find a heterogeneous terrain shaped by genetic factors, external conditions, and the fine tuning of internal mechanisms.

In this context, diabetes manifests itself in various forms: Type 1, Type 2, and gestational diabetes, each of which has its own set of difficulties and factors to take into account. The boundaries of this health domain are shaped by familial patterns and predispositions that are a result of the genetic foundations, which add another layer.

The terrain of diabetes is further shaped by environmental factors, such as lifestyle decisions and outside circumstances. There is a dynamic interaction between stress, physical activity, and diet. contribute to the undulating terrain of blood sugar levels.

Diabetes wellness: Customized diet solutions

Getting around this terrain requires identifying the subtle symptoms and signs that act as markers and point people in the direction of a clear diagnosis. Blood sugar levels fluctuate like the undulating hills and valleys of the terrain, necessitating a sophisticated comprehension of the effects of prescription drugs, way of life decisions, and food habits.

However, there are hills of wellness to be reached in this complicated terrain—holistic peaks that transcend simple blood sugar control. The broader picture of diabetes care includes cardiovascular health, mental health, and long-term problem prevention.

Using effective management techniques becomes essential for navigating this unstable environment. Personalized treatments, lifestyle changes, and the critical role that nutrition plays are all examples of adaptive approaches that enable people to manage their diabetes with resilience and confidence.

CHAPTER TWO

FOUNDATIONS OF DIABETES NUTRITION

A sophisticated comprehension of the effects of food choices on blood sugar levels, general health, and well-being forms the basis of diabetes nutrition. It encompasses several key concepts.

Proper Distribution of Macro-nutrients: Dietary practices for diabetes place a strong emphasis on consuming carbohydrates, proteins, and fats in a balanced manner. It is essential to comprehend how each macro-nutrient influences blood sugar levels in order to maintain stability.

Awareness of Carbohydrates: Blood sugar levels are directly impacted by carbohydrates. Controlling the kind and amount of carbohydrates is crucial. Making complex carbs—found in whole grains, fruits, and vegetables—a priority can help to maintain stable blood sugar levels and provide long-lasting energy.

Portion moderation: Keeping blood sugar levels from sharply fluctuating and regulating calorie intake are two benefits of portion control. A steady balance throughout the day is facilitated by portion sizes that are consistent.

Fiber-Rich Foods: When it comes to diabetes nutrition, foods high in dietary fiber—like fruits, vegetables, and whole grains—are essential. Fiber promotes digestive health and aids in blood sugar regulation.

Strategic Protein Intake: Consuming lean protein sources, like fish, poultry, legumes, and tofu, helps control blood sugar levels and promotes satiety.

Good Fats: Giving priority to foods high in good fats, like avocados, almonds, seeds, and olive oil, helps to maintain cardiovascular health. Additionally, these fats give meals more flavor and satisfaction.

Considerate Meal Planning: Eating at regular times helps control blood sugar levels. Steer clear of long intervals between meals to avoid severe swings and to encourage steady hypoglycemic control.

Individualized Approach: Taking into account cultural norms, personal preferences, and health objectives, an individualized approach acknowledges that every person has unique nutritional needs. Tailoring meal plans increases compliance and satisfaction.

Frequent Blood Sugar Monitoring: Keeping an eye on blood sugar levels on a regular basis offers important insights into how dietary decisions affect hypoglycemic management. Aware decision-making and adjustments are made possible by this awareness.

Cooperation with Medical Professionals: Consulting medical professionals, especially registered dietitians with expertise in diabetes management, guarantees a thorough and customized nutrition plan. Having professional assistance is important for long-term success when using nutrition to manage diabetes.

Diabetes wellness: Customized diet solutions

CHAPTER THREE

PERSONALIZED DIET APPROACHES

The customized diet approach is based on an approach that is specific to each person, taking into account their unique needs, preferences, and health goals. Rather than providing general dietary recommendations, this approach creates recommendations that take particular physiological, cultural, and lifestyle factors into account.

Fundamentally, a customized diet considers each person's specific nutritional needs while also incorporating knowledge from genetics to comprehend how a person's genetic makeup may affect how they react to particular foods. When it comes to creating dietary recommendations that support blood sugar control, weight management, or the special nutritional requirements for managing chronic conditions, health goals and conditions play a crucial role.

Culinary and cultural preferences are important because they honor the variety of influences and tastes that influence eating habits.

When customizing the diet plan, lifestyle factors like work schedules and physical activity are taken into account. This

Diabetes wellness: Customized diet solutions

method takes allergies and dietary sensitivities into account, guaranteeing enjoyment and security.

Furthermore, knowing a person's behavioral patterns makes it possible to design a personalized, long-lasting diet regimen. Regular monitoring and adjustments are part of the ongoing process, which recognizes that circumstances and nutritional needs can change over time.

This strategy has numerous advantages. Since the diet is more sustainable and fits with individual preferences, improved adherence is probably in store. Targeted nutrient absorption takes individual physiological variances into account. The strategy seeks to achieve particular health goals, such as better blood sugar regulation, weight loss, or increased energy. A person's personalized diet can become a useful and long-lasting aspect of their everyday routine by helping them develop a positive relationship with food and integrating it seamlessly with their lifestyle.

Essentially, the customized diet approach represents a break from general guidelines, acknowledging that optimal nutrition is a very personal journey.

CHAPTER FOUR

SUPER-FOODS FOR DIABETES

Super-foods are important dietary choices for people with diabetes because they provide a multitude of nutritional advantages beyond simple sustenance. The abundance of vitamins, minerals, antioxidants, and other bio-active substances that support general health are what define these nutrient-dense foods. Here are a few notable super-foods that are beneficial for people with diabetes:

Berries: Berries are a great source of fiber and antioxidants. Some examples of berries are blueberries, strawberries, and raspberries. Both blood sugar stabilization and inflammation reduction are facilitated by these compounds.

Fatty Fish: Omega-3 fatty acids are widely found in fatty fish, including mackerel and salmon. These heart-healthy fats have been linked to better cardiovascular and insulin sensitivity.

Leafy Greens: Rich in nutrients, dark greens such as kale and spinach are a nutrient powerhouse. They are high in fiber, vitamins, and minerals and provide a low-carb alternative for blood sugar regulation.

Nuts and Seeds: Rich in protein, fiber, and good fats, almonds, walnuts, chia seeds, and flax-seeds are nutrient-

Diabetes wellness: Customized diet solutions

dense options. They support stable blood sugar levels and satiety.

Whole Grains: Whole grains offer fiber and complex carbohydrates, like quinoa and oats. These grains provide steady energy because of their gradual effect on blood sugar.

Greek Yogurt: Rich in protein, Greek yogurt helps promote fullness and may be good for your gut because it contains macrobiotics.

Avocado: Packed with fiber and monounsaturated fats, avocados are low in blood sugar and a great source of many important nutrients.

Legumes: Rich in fiber, vitamins, and minerals, beans, lentils, and chickpeas are plant-based protein sources. Their effects on blood sugar and general metabolic health are positive.

Cinnamon: Adding cinnamon to food can add flavor and it's known to improve insulin sensitivity.

Turmeric: When added to the diet, turmeric, which contains cur-cumin, an anti-inflammatory compound, may have health benefits.

These super-foods can help with diabetes management and general well-being when added to a varied and balanced diet and when consulted by medical professionals or registered dietitians.

CHAPTER FIVE

MANAGING BLOOD SUGAR LEVELS

Maintaining optimal health requires effective blood sugar management, especially for those who have diabetes. This project is a complex commitment that extends beyond simple glucose management; it includes dietary decisions, consistent tracking, and a wholistic outlook on health.

The foundation of blood sugar control is dietary awareness. Stable blood sugar levels can be achieved by selecting nutrient-dense foods and placing an emphasis on whole grains, lean proteins, and healthy fats while also paying attention to portion sizes. It is important to be aware of carbohydrates and how different kinds of carbohydrates affect blood sugar.

One effective strategy for controlling blood sugar is physical activity. Frequent exercise promotes weight management, cardiovascular health, and improved insulin sensitivity. Fun activities are a great way to improve your physical and metabolic health on a daily basis.

Diabetes wellness: Customized diet solutions

One of the most important aspects of blood sugar control is following prescription drug regimens, when necessary. Timely and regular medication administration reduces the chance of problems and aids in maintaining stable glucose control.

In order to control blood sugar levels, stress management is essential. Because stress hormones can affect blood sugar levels, it's critical to include relaxation methods like deep breathing, mindfulness, or meditation in daily routines.

Frequent monitoring offers important information about how lifestyle decisions affect blood sugar levels. Making well-informed decisions enables prompt modifications to dietary practices, exercise routines, and medication schedules.

Frequently disregarded, hydration is essential for general well-being, including controlling blood sugar levels. Choosing water over sugar-filled drinks is a smart way to manage your diabetes.

Getting enough sleep is essential for maintaining good metabolic health. Making good sleep a priority enhances general well-being and improves insulin sensitivity.

Not only does weight control affect appearance, but it also has a big impact on blood sugar regulation. Reducing the risk of complications and improving insulin sensitivity are two benefits of reaching and maintaining a healthy weight.

Frequent medical examinations offer a thorough assessment of one's health. Tracking important metrics, like HbA1c levels, aids in evaluating long-term hypoglycemic control and directs changes to the management strategy.

Ongoing education gives you power. Keeping up with the most recent advancements in diabetes care, dietary recommendations, and lifestyle advice guarantees that people are prepared to make educated decisions regarding their health.

Essentially, controlling blood sugar is a dynamic, all-encompassing commitment to well-being rather than a single task. It entails adopting a healthy lifestyle, making well-informed decisions, and developing cooperative relationships with medical professionals. Through these initiatives, people can manage their diabetes with resiliency and a goal of attaining long-term health and vitality.

Diabetes wellness: Customized diet solutions

CHAPTER SIX

CUSTOMIZING YOUR PLATE

Making a plate that reflects your unique dietary requirements and preferences is a deeply personal and liberating experience. Creating a personalized meal plan entails taking into account the nutrients your body needs and your own personal culinary preferences.

Start by realizing how crucial it is to have a balanced diet. Try to consume a balance of fats, proteins, and carbohydrates to give your body the nutrition and energy it needs to operate at its best. Pick a range of vibrantly colored fruits and vegetables for their varied range of vitamins and minerals, in addition to their vibrant flavors.

Remaining within a healthy weight range and avoiding overindulgence in food require mindful portion control. Pay attention to your body's signals of hunger and fullness, and take time to enjoy every taste.

Lean protein sources, such as fish, poultry, tofu, and legumes, can support healthy muscles and general well-being. Whole grains provide a healthy base for your meals by supplying vital nutrients and fiber, like brown rice and quinoa.

Diabetes wellness: Customized diet solutions

Include foods high in healthy fats, such as nuts and avocados, to promote satiety and a range of body functions. For the sake of your general health and digestion, always remember to drink water with your meals as hydration is equally important.

Explore your creativity when it comes to cooking by experimenting with herbs and spices. This enhances the flavor of your food and offers further health advantages. Customizing your plate should take your unique requirements and tastes into account. Personal preferences, cultural influences, or dietary restrictions—customizing your meals guarantees that they fit your particular way of life.

Lastly, learn to embrace intuitive eating. Eat with awareness and enjoy the flavors and textures of your food. A healthy relationship with food can be developed that benefits your general well-being by listening to your body's cues and savoring the act of eating.

CHAPTER SEVEN

BEYOND DIET - LIFESTYLE CHANGES

Setting out on a path that extends beyond simple dietary decisions, lifestyle modifications refer to an all-encompassing metamorphosis that includes mental, emotional, and physical health. It goes beyond the traditional idea of a diet as a temporary solution and becomes a long-term dedication to general health and vitality.

In terms of nutrition, the goal is to shift the emphasis from calorie counting to foods high in nutrients that provide the body with nourishment. Whole, unprocessed foods high in vital vitamins, minerals, and antioxidants are emphasized because they support resilience against health challenges and help with weight management.

Exercise takes center stage as a source of energy, better cardiovascular health, and improved mental well-being rather than just as a means of burning calories. Sustainable lifestyle adjustments place a higher priority on joyful and fulfilling physical activity, promoting a lasting commitment to movement.

Diabetes wellness: Customized diet solutions

Eating with awareness turns into a tenet that encourages people to relish every bite of their food. By encouraging a deeper connection with the act of nourishment and avoiding emotional or mindless eating, this practice cultivates a positive relationship with food.

The change in lifestyle goes beyond the physical to include stress reduction and emotional health. Understanding the detrimental effects of stress on one's health, people incorporate techniques like deep breathing, meditation, or hobby-playing to build emotional resilience.

A vital element is quality sleep, with people placing a high value on getting enough rest to recover. Sufficient sleep promotes overall health by influencing hormone balance, mental clarity, and emotional stability.
Creating habits that are supportive becomes essential to the lifestyle shift. The cornerstones of long-term health include eating at regular times, drinking plenty of water, and creating a happy atmosphere at work and home.

A dedication to ongoing education and flexibility defines the path beyond nutrition. Having up-to-date knowledge about wellness, nutrition, and new research enables people to make wise decisions and modify their lifestyles to suit changing needs.

Significantly, the emphasis moves from quick fixes to long-term, sustainable decisions. Not only is immediate efficacy desired, but long-term habits that promote health all through life are also desired.

Adopting a lifestyle that goes beyond diet is essentially a call to a lasting and transformative journey. It entails a comprehensive dedication to providing the body with nourishment, practicing mindfulness, promoting mental health, and creating enduring habits. Beyond food, there is a significant chance for people to develop a vibrant, balanced, and long-lasting well-being-filled life.

Diabetes wellness: Customized diet solutions

CHAPTER EIGHT

SPECIAL CONSIDERATIONS FOR DIABETES COMPLICATIONS

A keen eye for potential complications is necessary when navigating the complicated terrain of diabetes, with particular attention paid to heart health, kidney function, and eye care. People managing their diabetes must take a proactive and nuanced approach in these three crucial areas.

- Heart Health

Heart health is extremely important because diabetics have a higher risk of heart disease. Important things to think about are:

Blood Pressure Management: In order to keep blood pressure levels in a healthy range, lifestyle modifications, regular monitoring, and prescribed medication are essential.

Control of Cholesterol: Lowering cardiovascular risks and controlling cholesterol levels can be achieved with a heart-healthy diet, frequent exercise, and adherence to prescription medicine.

Diabetes wellness: Customized diet solutions

Blood Sugar Regulation: One of the most important ways to avoid heart-related problems is to maintain consistent blood sugar control through diet and medication adherence.

- Kidney Function

Since diabetes is a major risk factor for developing chronic kidney disease, kidney health must be protected proactively. Important tactics consist of:

Blood Pressure Regulation: The key to avoiding kidney problems is controlling blood pressure with medication and lifestyle changes.

Frequent evaluations of kidney function, such as serum creatinine and urine albumin tests, offer valuable information about kidney health and facilitate timely intervention.

Optimal Blood Sugar Management: Kidney damage can be prevented by maintaining stable blood sugar levels, which can be attained by following prescription instructions and making lifestyle changes.

Dr. Harmony Wells

Diabetes wellness: Customized diet solutions

- Eye Care

Because diabetic retinopathy is a serious risk to vision, it is imperative that you take great care of your eyes.

Frequent Eye Exams: To prevent or treat diabetic nephropathy, yearly thorough eye exams are necessary for early detection and prompt intervention.

Blood Sugar Stability: Maintaining general eye health and lowering the risk of diabetic nephropathy require regular blood sugar management.

Blood Pressure Control: To maintain the best possible eye health, regular monitoring and a heart-healthy lifestyle are important.

In summary, a holistic strategy for managing diabetes involves not only regular blood sugar regulation but also heart health, kidney function, and eye care. People can reduce the risk of complications and improve their general well-being by taking a proactive approach that includes routine monitoring, lifestyle modifications, and adherence to prescribed medications. Having regular conversations with medical specialists is still essential to developing a customized and successful diabetes care plan.

Dr. Harmony Wells

Diabetes wellness: Customized diet solutions

Diabetes wellness: Customized diet solutions

CHAPTER NINE

COOKING FOR DIABETES WELLNESS

When it comes to diabetes management, the kitchen becomes an infinite resource, providing a blank canvas for imagination and a place to nourish the body and the soul. Cooking for diabetes wellness is more than just putting food on the table; it's a holistic process that combines culinary artistry and nutritional knowledge.

This culinary approach's fundamental idea is balanced nutrition. The meals are a tapestry of nutrient-dense foods, ranging from lean proteins and whole grains to healthy fats and a rainbow of vibrant fruits and vegetables. The palate turns into a symphony of flavors that harmonize to provide the body with complete nourishment.

The focus is on mindful management of carbohydrates, which encourages a sophisticated understanding of the different kinds of carbohydrates ingested. Complex, slowly-releasing foods like sweet potatoes and quinoa become mainstays, their measured presence helping to maintain a stable blood sugar balance. Controlling portion sizes becomes an attentive exercise that follows your body's natural wisdom.

Diabetes wellness: Customized diet solutions

Plant-based proteins come to life as colorful heroes who not only offer vital nutrients but also give the culinary story more nuance. On the plate, legumes, tofu, and tempeh support long-term energy and general health. The movement toward plant-based cuisine aligns with both a growing environmental consciousness and dietary sensitivities.
When healthy fats are included, it becomes an artistic endeavor, with avocados, nuts, seeds, and olive oil serving as storytellers of richness and satiety rather than just being ingredients. The skill is in striking the right balance between gastronomic pleasure and health awareness.

Spices and herbs take center stage, acting not just as flavor enhancers but also as main characters on their own. In addition to enhancing the flavor of food, spices like turmeric, basil, and cilantro may also have health advantages. The kitchen transforms into a flavor laboratory that encourages experimentation and ingenuity.

Portion control is no longer just about numbers; it has become a conscious, intuitive eating technique. Plate design that balances carbs, proteins, and fats becomes a skill for controlling blood sugar and promoting a closer bond with the act of eating.

The kitchen becomes an experimental space where recipe modification becomes a creative expression. Reducing sugar content, embracing high-fiber options, and using alternative ingredients become paintbrush strokes on the culinary canvas. This artistic investigation aims to redefine what is achievable in the kitchen rather than merely modify recipes.

Meal preparation becomes a self-care ritual rather than a practicality. It entails developing a well-balanced repertory, exploring flavors, and giving careful thought to nutritional requirements. When food is prepared in bulk, it becomes a celebration of nourishment, with meal preparation becoming just as important as meal consumption.

Hydration becomes more important than just a basic biological requirement. Water is now the main drink, along with herbal teas and other infused drinks. The focus on beverages aligns not just with quenching thirst but with contributing to overall well-being.

Eating turns into a festivity and goes beyond just ingesting food. Creating a warm environment, appreciating every taste, and encouraging a healthy relationship with food become essential components of the experience. It's a recognition that eating well is just as important to overall wellness as diet.

Diabetes wellness: Customized diet solutions

Cooking to promote diabetes wellness is an ongoing educational and exploratory process. Keeping up with dietary recommendations, experimenting with new dishes, and adjusting to changing preferences all play crucial roles in this dynamic story. It's an adventure that never stops changing and calls for both curiosity and flexibility.

Cooking for diabetes wellness is essentially a celebration of life through nourishment, rather than merely a means of managing a medical condition. It's a gastronomic journey that encourages people to interact with food in a way that not only effectively manages diabetes but also transforms the routine activities of preparing and eating meals into a comprehensive celebration of health.

CHAPTER TEN

NAVIGATING SOCIAL AND PRACTICAL CHALLENGES

A distinct set of social and practical challenges arises from having diabetes. Managing the illness well requires handling circumstances that go beyond routine blood sugar checks. Two important factors that need to be carefully considered are eating out and traveling while diabetic.

Eating Out: Managing diabetes becomes more difficult when dining at restaurants or at social events, but it is a challenge that can be overcome with careful planning and effective communication.

Strategic Menu Selection: Choose whole grains, lean proteins, and lots of vegetables when looking through a menu. Selecting baked, steamed, or grilled foods instead of fried ones can help reduce calorie intake and blood sugar levels.

Control Your Portion: Serving sizes at restaurants are frequently larger than what is advised. Think about asking to split a dish with a dining partner or requesting a smaller portion. Being mindful of portion control aids in managing blood sugar levels.

Communication with Staff: Don't be afraid to let restaurant staff know about any special needs or dietary preferences. A lot of places are friendly and will adjust meals to meet your requirements. You can be sure that the restaurant is diabetes-friendly by inquiring about preparation techniques and ingredient replacements.

Smart Carbohydrate Management: Exercise caution when consuming foods high in carbohydrates. Choose whole grains and ask about dressings and sauces' carbohydrate contents. Maintaining blood sugar stability is aided by balancing carbohydrate intake.

Traveling with Diabetes: People who have diabetes face additional logistical difficulties when they travel. To guarantee a smooth journey, awareness and preparation are essential.

Medication and Supplies: Make sure you have enough insulin, prescription drugs, and testing supplies with you. Bring extra in case there are unforeseen delays. To preserve their efficacy, make sure medications are stored correctly, particularly when traveling by air.

Healthy Snacks:

Have a stash of healthy snacks readily available. Unpredictable meal times during travel can lead to irregular eating patterns, and having nutritious snacks on hand helps stabilize blood sugar levels.

Hydration:

Stay well-hydrated, especially when flying, to prevent dehydration, a common concern for people with diabetes. Carry a refillable water bottle and avoid sugary drinks.

Time Zone Adjustments:

If crossing time zones, coordinate medication schedules with the new time zone. Consult with a healthcare professional to adjust dosages as needed.

Emergency Preparedness:

Be prepared for unexpected situations. Carry a medical identification card, a list of emergency contacts, and a brief explanation of your diabetes management plan. Familiarize yourself with local medical facilities at your destination.

Healthy Snacks: Always keep a supply of nutritious snacks on hand. Traveling with unpredictable meal times can cause irregular eating patterns; keeping wholesome snacks on hand can help stabilize blood sugar levels.

Diabetes wellness: Customized diet solutions

Hydration: Avoid dehydration, which is a common worry for diabetics, by drinking plenty of water, especially when flying. Avoid sugary drinks and always have a refillable water bottle with you.

Time Zone Changes: Make sure your medication schedules are adjusted to the new time zone when traveling across time zones. If necessary, seek advice from a healthcare provider to modify the dosage.

Emergency Readiness: Always be ready for unforeseen circumstances. Keep a list of emergency contacts, a medical identity card, and a brief description of your diabetes management strategy with you at all times. At your destination, familiarize yourself with the local medical facilities.

Frequent Blood Sugar Monitoring: Keep a regular blood sugar monitoring schedule. Variations in routine, like eating at different times or traveling at a higher level of activity, can affect blood sugar levels. Timely modifications are possible with regular monitoring.

Using a combination of proactive planning, good communication, and strategic decision-making, one can effectively navigate the social and practical challenges surrounding diabetes. People with diabetes can lead meaningful and enriching lives in addition to effectively managing their condition by adopting a thoughtful mindset when dining out and traveling. Frequent consultations with medical professionals can help foster a self-assured and empowered approach to diabetes management by offering customized guidance for particular circumstances.

Diabetes wellness: Customized diet solutions

CONCLUSION

EMPOWERING YOURSELF FOR DIABETES WELLNESS

To sum up, the path to diabetes wellness is an active and liberating one. Beyond controlling blood sugar levels, it encompasses a comprehensive dedication to overall health. Developing a healthy relationship with food, adopting an active, balanced lifestyle, and taking proactive measures to overcome social and practical obstacles are all part of empowering yourself for diabetes wellness.

Making educated nutritional decisions, engaging in regular physical activity, and communicating effectively with healthcare providers are essential elements of this empowerment. Having the understanding that managing diabetes is an ongoing learning process promotes resilience and adaptability.People who approach life's challenges with a proactive mentality can not only successfully manage their illness but also succeed in living a full and active life.

Recall that empowerment is realizing how every decision affects one's general state of well-being. Every step on the path to diabetes wellness is a monument to the fortitude and resiliency that come with it, whether it be choosing food wisely, exercising frequently, or interacting confidently in social settings. People who feel empowered are able to take control of their health and make decisions that will result in a full and active life.